What I Wished I Knew 30 Years Ago

What I Wished I Knew 30 Years Ago

Bipolar Mixed Mood

Sarah Andrews

Copyright © 2020 by Sarah Andrews.

Library of Congress Control Number:		2020903423
ISBN:	Hardcover	978-1-5434-9618-5
	Softcover	978-1-5434-9617-8
	eBook	978-1-5434-9616-1

All rights reserved. No part of this book may be reproduced or transmitted in any form or by any means, electronic or mechanical, including photocopying, recording, or by any information storage and retrieval system, without permission in writing from the copyright owner.

Any people depicted in stock imagery provided by Getty Images are models, and such images are being used for illustrative purposes only.
Certain stock imagery © Getty Images.

Print information available on the last page.

Rev. date: 02/24/2020

To order additional copies of this book, contact:
Xlibris
0-800-443-678
www.Xlibris.co.nz
Orders@Xlibris.co.nz

CONTENTS

Introduction vii

Chapter 1   Getting to Grips with the Public Mental Health System ... 1
Chapter 2   Timeline of Nicola's Diagnosis 4
Chapter 3   What Is Bipolar Mixed Mood? 7
Chapter 4   When it All Began 9
Chapter 5   First Appointment with a Private Psychiatrist on
            4 August 1995 12
Chapter 6   Nicola's Story: The Visit 15
Chapter 7   More Chaos 19
Chapter 8   A Mixed State 22
Chapter 9   Two Days in the Life of Nicola 25
Chapter 10 Second Opinion 30
Chapter 11 Some Headway 33
Chapter 12 An Evening Walk 36
Chapter 13 Stigma 38
Chapter 14 Plagued by Diagnosis 41
Chapter 15 Post-Traumatic Stress Disorder (PTSD) 44
Chapter 16 You Can Heal and Recover from the Effects of
            Trauma 47
Chapter 17 Obstructive Sleep Apnoea 50

Chapter 18 Moving to the Public Mental Health Services
            and Specialist Hospital..54
Chapter 19 At the Specialist Hospital..57
Chapter 20 Crazy Mental Health Assistance 59
Chapter 21 Metabolic Monitoring of Antipsychotic Medication.....61
Chapter 22 What Is Treatment Resistance in Psychiatry?..............64
Chapter 23 Rapid Metabolizer 67
Chapter 24 Final Thoughts on What We Could Do Better............72

Appendix 75
References 77

INTRODUCTION

This book contains the experiences and views of the author and is shared with the understanding that the author is not providing professional advice. Many of the names and details of individuals have been changed to protect their privacy and reputation, including the name of my daughter.

Bipolar disorder is a severe mood disorder, a malignant and deadly disease which affects 2.6 per cent of the population, or 60 million worldwide.

Because I have been a caregiver/parent to a person suffering from a subtype of bipolar disorder (mixed state), I have written this book about the knowledge I have accumulated over the past twenty-nine years. There have been unique challenges and complex issues I faced as a caregiver. Before we had the Internet, research about bipolar disorder could only be obtained through reading, speaking to professionals, or through networking with other caregivers. This information often did not match up with what I was experiencing with my daughter. From the time that Nicola was about twelve years old, it became almost a full-time occupation for me, as her mother, to puzzle out her perplexing behaviour. It is interesting that nearly three decades have passed, and there is still not a single book or memoir on the mixed state of bipolar disorder that a lay person could read. I have tried to write the book that I would have loved to read all those years ago. I remember reading pages from medical books I found in the library and trying to match Nicola's behaviour to different diagnoses that had been suggested by doctors, such as chronic fatigue syndrome or glandular fever or teenage bad behaviour. Nothing ever corresponded, which fuelled my exasperation. By writing this book, with its vignettes, I am outlining the journey it took for us to get an accurate diagnosis, to be provided treatment in the form of medication and psychotherapy, and to finally locate the missing key factors that contributed to recovery.

I hope this book will save years of anguish and despondency for caregivers and sufferers, and give hope and encouragement to all those who are bravely involved with this disorder.

CHAPTER 1

Getting to Grips with the Public Mental Health System

I was about to enter a protracted nightmare. I was woefully underprepared for my role as a caregiver and for the medical and nursing responsibilities I was asked and expected to perform. There was no caregiver's handbook, but I imagined that this would be only for a short period, maybe a couple of months once the medication started working its magic. I could never have foreseen that this role would go on for decades.

Over thirty years, I would develop my own areas of expertise. I would come to learn the names of hundreds of drugs with their side effects, half-lives, withdrawal symptoms, doses, and interactions; encounter heaps of disorders with similar symptoms; and personally meet those individuals with these symptoms. I gleaned what I could from the clinical staff, with their specialized knowledge, and refuted what I considered rubbish.

Apart from when Nicola was in the hospital, I had no idea as to what my function was to be in managing her day-to-day life. In all those years of her illness, I went on blindly, eventually learning the procedures that enabled Nicola to receive different kinds of treatment for her mental illness. Over the thirty years that I struggled to master the system, I realized that I was so keen to get Nicola well that I was doing her a huge disservice, micromanaging her. I was doing her tasks, which downplayed her illness to the professionals. And so of course, how could clinical staff realize the full impact of her illness?

If she had lived on her own, missed appointments, and led a messy, disorganized life, her behaviour would have resulted in police action. Then she would have had more clinical attention, maybe a compulsory treatment order and more time in a ward for observation. I had spent so much time shielding her from the realities, hovering and being the perfect co-dependent.

James Aiken (2017), page 278, quotes Dr Akiskal (2011) in saying 'it is often the mother who carries the brunt of the illness' burden [in bipolar]'. Aiken (2017) also adds that 'mothers carry a strong sense of responsibility for their children and may blame themselves for the problem. They don't need extra help with that guilt, but that doesn't stop other people from lending an unhelpful hand. If she is supportive and nurturing, she's accused of enabling the illness; if she steps back, she's cold and neglectful.'

I imagine that very few patients have an advocate that is ready to act when life became too abysmal for the patient. Along the way, I was constantly questioning myself about how assertive I needed to be before I was viewed as overbearing. Could I really trust that I was getting the correct advice from a twenty-three-year-old nurse or occupational therapist? I experienced a wide variation in responses from staff. Some would placate and be totally ineffective while others would become a controlling parent determined to keep both patient and parent firmly in their place.

A lot of rules were kept obscure. How much easier it would have been to just have a pamphlet outlining how to get a prescription, how to access a psychiatrist, the role of a nurse, the role of receptionist, what to do if your key worker is unavailable, at what stage do you visit the ED . . . Something else I learned was a special protocol to deliver messages and rules about staff hierarchy. I learned to accept that it may be days or weeks to get advice when things went wrong. Sometimes, at the risk of being chastised by nurses or psychiatrists, I had to make my own decisions about issues.

Every general practitioner (GP) I spoke to in the interim was amazingly helpful even though they had had very limited training in this area, and I had to clue them in on some new information that I had learned. There were times when I found it hard to get an urgent appointment with a GP. I was persistent when the receptionist asked why I wanted an appointment and could not understand why I was so insistent, since my daughter's problem was only insomnia. She could not comprehend that this symptom could be the beginning of a slippery slope for some patients.

Then I found the private system. How lovely to sit and be intently listened to and validated by a respectful professional. If you have the money, you can have as many sessions as you need and be able to pick and choose your appointment times and try out who may be able to address your needs. You may even have access to email or direct phone calls. To lessen the pain of these appointments, I found it wise to choose the least defensive person. By interviewing doctors, it quickly became apparent who these were. To spare Nicola extra stress, I wanted to do the groundwork for her. One bonus was they did not move on after three or six months, as would happen in the public system. I have never been shouted at or chastised by a private psychiatrist. The only downfall I came across was they were not able to treat a patient with Clozapine. This was restricted to the first two years of treatment within a public hospital, as it needed to be monitored carefully by an outside drug company. Although they had contacts with clinical psychologists, they often did not have contacts such as a social worker or occupational therapist or nurse.

My role as a caregiver covered three decades. In the final year, everything became manageable, even exciting, as I witnessed Nicola's progress in the art of living life become a satisfying adventure. It was at the end of the third decade that the missing piece to the puzzle was found, and I owe this to two psychiatrists who courageously followed their convictions.

CHAPTER 2

Timeline of Nicola's Diagnosis

It is usually best to start with getting to know the disorder intimately. The more information you have about the disorder, the better equipped you'll be to handle the next move. The following ideas came from the website www.bphope.com/history-of-bipolar.

By looking at a brief timeline, you can see how the term *bipolar disorder* originated from the term *manic depression*. The ancient Greeks and Romans came up with the terms *melancholia* and *mania*. In 1851 a French psychiatrist, Fairet, described a condition *la folie circulaire*, which translates to 'circular insanity'. He documented people switching through depression and mania, and noted genetic connections. Kraepelin, in 1921, differentiated the difference between manic depression and praecox (schizophrenia), and this classification of mental disorders became part of the basis for the manual *DSM-5* used by psychiatrists today. The term *bipolar disorder* appeared in the *DSM-III* in 1980 to avoid calling patients 'maniacs'.

The *DSM-5* is the most recent edition (2013) of the book, which is the bible for psychologists and psychiatrists in New Zealand and elsewhere. The initials stand for *Diagnostic and Statistical Manual of Mental Disorders*. It is the definitive guide for patterns of behaviour and their treatment. What is, and what is not, contained in the *DSM* through each of its revisions is the source of much argument amongst professionals. This latest *DSM-5* now includes bipolar, with mixed features (which is both depression and mania occurring together), and it is especially prevalent in younger patients.

Over the course of twenty-nine years, Nicola saw many psychiatrists, many of whom could not agree on her diagnosis. As a result, Nicola received numerous treatments, none of which were effective. In 2018, a treatment rarely used in New Zealand for bipolar seemed to be promising. It was implemented by a plucky female psychiatrist and came close to hitting the jackpot, but not quite. The turning point was to come with further insight and another drug to increase the bioavailability of the current medication, again by another forward-thinking female psychiatrist.

When Nicola first became unwell three decades ago, the term *bipolar* was frequently called *manic depression*. This contributed to the lack of knowledge by professionals on the mixed states condition. It was also thought that young people could not even have bipolar. The first psychiatrist my daughter saw in 1995, referred to it as possible manic depression. Then he discounted it because her symptoms didn't match the current *DSM* and decided that it was a behaviour problem. Although some children meet the criteria, many fall outside these classical categories, and diagnosis in these children is particularly challenging and difficult. Nicola had symptoms every single day, unlike adult bipolar, which can have gaps between mood switches.

The next doctor, a child and adolescent psychiatrist, thought it was the adolescent variety of bipolar, after hearing Barbara Geller speak at a conference about childhood bipolar and how it was the most severe kind and often misdiagnosed. Unfortunately, this diagnosis was thrown out the window after two more psychiatrists thought it was borderline personality disorder or cyclothymia. The mixed-mood diagnosis was finally reinstated in 2010 and finally treated appropriately in 2019, thirty years after Nicola's initial symptoms appeared. During those times, Nicola saw many clinicians, most of whom were doing their best to be supportive. She saw ten different GPs, seven counsellors, four clinical psychologists, eleven consultant psychiatrists, four registrars, four occupational therapists, and dozens of nurses. One hospital cleaner declared she was just in a shitty mood. Nicola listened to all their advice, but no progress was ever made, and as is the nature of bipolar if untreated, her condition worsened. Treatment is very necessary to protect against the deterioration associated with repeated acute episodes. For all the progress made, or lack of it, I sometimes cynically thought I may as well have consulted our neighbours or the postman and made just as much progress. Fortunately, in 2018 and 2019 we met two incredible advocates, and the last pieces to the puzzle were found. This led to a successful recovery.

CHAPTER 3

What Is Bipolar Mixed Mood?

I had never heard of this phenomenon called bipolar disorder and given that approximately 2.6 per cent of adults in the Western world have this disorder (formally called manic depression) it is surprising that I hadn't. There are no medical tests to diagnose bipolar disorder, and there is no single cause for bipolar disorder. It is a complex condition with many contributing factors, which can include neurotransmitters, serotonin and dopamine functioning improperly, and/or genetics. The *DSM-5* (2013) has reported that there is an average '10-fold increased risk among adult relatives with bipolar I and bipolar II disorders'. In Nicola's case, I researched and found that there were several generations of relatives affected, two of whom committed suicide. One had schizoaffective, and the other had involutional melancholia. Outside factors, such as stress or a major life event, may trigger a genetic predisposition or potential biological reaction, but medical researchers have still not yet identified the causes and its presentations.

What I learned was that there are different types of bipolar disorder.

Bipolar I is considered the classic type, where individuals experience both manic and depressive episodes of varying lengths.

Bipolar II involves less severe manic episodes than bipolar I; however, their depressive episodes are the same.

Cyclothymia is a chronic but milder form of bipolar disorder.

Mixed episodes are where both mania and depression occur simultaneously. Some state that an estimated 40 per cent of people who live with bipolar disorder experience mixed symptoms, but it is grossly under-recognized.

Rapid cycling is where individuals experience four or more episodes of mania, depression, or both within one year.

It was the mixed affective state that was to dominate Nicola's life, and it was present every day of her life.

A mixed affective state, formally known as a mixed episode, is defined as a state wherein both depression and mania occur either simultaneously or in very short succession. Unfortunately, the ups and downs don't cancel each other out; rather, the overlap causes anxiety and tension as the symptoms pull in opposite directions. The term *bipolar* does not capture the experience of a mixed state. The hallmarks of a mixed state comprise agitation, anxiety, insomnia, lack of concentration, and extreme irritability. You can be sarcastic, demanding, and have no patience. Your sleeping pattern could be 6 a.m.–4 p.m. or no sleep at all for days. The anxiety part leads people to hurt themselves, break things, or lash out at people.

A person with mixed features might appear to feel euphoric while crying or may experience a rush of thoughts while also in a state of lethargy. The thing I didn't understand at that point was how readily mixed state bipolar could be fatal. The risk of suicide or potential harm to another person is high. I have been told that 60 per cent of bipolar patients attempt suicide, and 30 per cent are successful. Combined with impulsivity, it is a dangerous condition. For the patient, it is an unbearable state to be in. I thought we were fighting for the quality of her life, not her survival, and this became the beginning of many unexpected and challenging experiences that lay ahead.

CHAPTER 4

When it All Began

It is hard to pinpoint exactly when subtle emotional changes in my typically calm and pleasant daughter became exaggeratedly abnormal. It did not appear to be the usual vagaries of adolescence such as anxiety from peer pressure. Rather she started to be unable to organise herself before school. She was only required to put on her school uniform, eat breakfast and get in the car, to be driven the ten kilometres to school. Considering she had no chores, no siblings to hassle her and no lunch to prepare, one would think that this could be accomplished in 30 minutes. But this routine could take Nicola hours.

It would start with some disquiet which would then accelerate to a fretting, and full-on frustration attack. This all concerned her hair. Her anxiety over her hair affected her so much that 2 hours could pass and even then, it could not be completed to her satisfaction. In desperation after experimenting with reassurance and setting a time limit, I came up with the idea that peer pressure or shaming might spur her on, so I called on the assistance of a baffled school friend. It made no difference and eventually exasperated, I would drag her to the car as she clutched her collection of brushes, combs and clips. On the whole drive to school she would be peering into the visor mirror, twisting, flattening, positioning locks of hair, followed with more smoothing out. Then with great frustration she would start it all over again. By this time, we were at the school gates and I had to shove her out through the car door. It all seemed very peculiar as just six months prior, she was Miss Efficiency herself, to the point that when I went overseas for six weeks, she thrived, enjoying her independence at home with her father. I started to wonder if she had some type of obsessive-compulsive disorder. The hair episode lasted most of that year and then suddenly disappeared.

What appeared to take its place was a reluctance to get out of bed in the morning. For a girl with many friends and good school results it was a puzzle. When quizzed, she said she felt very tired. After a few days of her staring at the ceiling I took her to our GP. He wondered if it was glandular fever but that proved negative. Another week went by and back to the GP who then thought it was a kind of chronic fatigue syndrome or Tapanui Flu as it was known in New Zealand. He suggested an appointment with the Child and Family Clinic but there was a long waiting list of ten weeks. He prescribed 75mg of Prothiaden, an old-style antidepressant, in the meantime.

At this time, she appeared to be having fluctuations in her mood. The longest that an extremely low mood lasted was four days. She said this low mood was the worst feeling she had ever had, and she felt a failure, and so guilty for causing trouble. She would pick flowers for me, to make me feel better. During one of these episodes she said she felt so shocking she thought she would "fall off the world". One day she started to cut her wrist but went no further than a scratch. At this time, she started to store knives under her bed and grab pills. When she got very low, she thought it would be easier to be dead.

Then would come a mood where she felt motivated and inspired to do lots of schoolwork. Each night she would write a list about what was required for her to do to get ready for school and how many minutes would be allocated to each task. She often would not get past the first item.

Getting sleep at night was an enormous problem. When Nicola took hours to get to sleep, she would regularly make a trip to our room to inform us. This could be every hour until about 4am. I grew to dread the warning squeak of the door from her bedroom, as she came in.

There were also times when she would become enraged. There was never a trigger. I was perturbed about how much school she was missing so I contacted a psychiatrist who worked in a private capacity. This was organised in two days and I grew very hopeful that this problem would be swiftly dealt with.

CHAPTER 5

First Appointment with a Private Psychiatrist on 4 August 1995

Nicola's father and I accompanied Nicola to an evening appointment at a medical centre in a town near us. Nicola was eager to get her problem solved, and we hoped that it would resolve this matter enough, so we could get back to an ordinary life. We gauged that the cost of $240 was fair enough for a complete cure.

However, from the moment Nicola, her father, and I entered the psychiatrist's room, Nicola was uncooperative. She refused to shake his hand and at first resented his questioning, answering some with a surly shake of her head. With a little prompting by me, she contributed a little to the history, such as sleep problems and the blood tests (which were all normal) and her various emotions of anger and feeling down.

The psychiatrist then launched an attack in what I presumed was his version of family therapy.

'What's been going on between you?' he snarled, looking at me and my husband. My husband looked startled, and I groaned inwardly. It was not an encouraging start for him, who believed there was no problem, and so was reluctant to even attend the appointment.

The 'family therapy' focused on the problem of Nicola missing a lot of school because she had insomnia and hence slept in too late the next morning. By the end of the session, the psychiatrist came up with a plan. We parents were to go into her bedroom holding hands and order her out of bed. Double the power, I suppose. We then left with a prescription for Prozac, with instructions to dissolve it in apple juice, and a pamphlet about the link of Prozac to suicide.

The next morning, we attempted to carry out the instructions. It failed, as each time we pulled her out of bed, she climbed back in, pulling her duvet up to her chin. We tried for several mornings, with her getting increasingly distressed. After a payment to the doctor equalling a week's wages for us, I felt we had made no progress at all.

And so, began a theme that would last for the next three decades. Endless driving to appointments, only to have hope dashed and to never find any solutions.

The next week was another appointment with the doctor. This time we left with a prescription for 2 mg Clonazepam, which was to prove ineffective. We tried his suggestion of Bach flowers, chamomile tea, and grounding exercises, but there was no improvement from these either.

He suggested that Nicola see a clinical psychologist. This proved to be a satisfactory experience for Nicola, who learned about sleep hygiene and self-hypnotic techniques. We felt that this was a positive move, but sadly, the sleep problem persisted.

A few days later, getting increasingly irritated at the no-sleep pattern, I ditched the professional's advice and focused on the local pharmacist's sleep remedies. Looking around the shelves, I spied some familiar items which all induced sleep—travel pills, teething medications, and antihistamines. I tried each one, but none had the slightest effect. Usually, around 4 a.m., after a rambunctious evening, she would drop off to sleep.

During the next consultation with the psychiatrist, which only I attended, he enlightened me with what his thoughts were. I scrambled to take notes, and this is the gist of it which I wrote out as soon as I got home. It was a good summary and coincided with what I thought.

> She is chronically tired and unable to concentrate. She feels very emotional and often tearful. She knows that she is good at her schoolwork but lacks motivation. She

admits she feels like a real failure and within a day can go up and down in mood. She lacks control over emotions and feels at times like giving up. She feels hopeless and powerless for the last two weeks that she has been off school. On one occasion she didn't get out of bed for three days. Last week she felt she couldn't go on and for the first time was thinking she wished she was dead. When she has fantasies of killing herself, everything seems too painful. She states that she doesn't want to kill herself because she in fact wants to get better and is determined to do so. She has no actual plan or action intended, as far as suicide is concerned. Although she gets angry with her mother, she has made a 'no self-harm' commitment to her. Her appetite is satisfactory with no eating disturbance. She gets frustrated at being awake with thoughts going over the past and future, and she would like to switch off all this thinking. In recent months, her mood has been worse in the morning and gradually picks up, particularly if she is around her friends at school who provide a distraction.

It is interesting to read Dr Barbara Geller, a psychiatry professor, and her views of how children do not have well periods, unlike adults who can have a high or low, with well patches in between. She says that a child can be manic and amusing, and a few minutes later, can be suicidal and talk about stabbing themselves in the heart. We were to see this repeatedly over the years.

At this time, I started to feel the backlash from friends and family as people became inconvenienced by Nicola's unpredictability. To them, the solution seemed simple: just stop being sick! They thought of her as lazy, attention-seeking, and weak-willed. This was reinforced when we needed to cancel plans, backed out at the last minute of an event, or failed to turn up to meet a friend. People were not forgiving, and this added further pressure. It was impossible for her to commit to arrangements, and no doubt, Nicola was thought of as too good for their company or just plain flaky and uninterested.

CHAPTER 6

Nicola's Story: The Visit

It was while Nicola was seeing her first psychiatrist that she became inspired to write. Suddenly, streams of poetry, clever rhyming ditties, stories, and letters to celebrities were carved out on scraps of paper. It became her bedroom wallpaper, and it seemed that there was no thinking process or planning beforehand. I have included one of her writings, which is a recount of her visit to a psychiatrist.

* * *

'What did you say his name was again?' I asked as I stared at a rip in the back of Mum's car seat.

'He is just a doctor.'

'How boring,' I said to pretend I didn't care.

Mum carried on driving, determined.

I remembered back to last night when she said, 'This outrageous behaviour has been going on for far too long!'

I focused on Mum's blue shoulder, avoiding her eyes at all costs.

'You are disrespectful and spiteful. We're sending you to a professional'.

My head was roaring with anger, but I pushed it aside to ask, 'A professional? Like whom? You know I don't mean to be this way!'

'I mean a psychiatrist.'

Mum parked behind a dark-green station wagon. We got out of the car and entered the building. We took a right turn up some carpeted steps to where the names of several psychiatrists, dieticians, and cardiologists were displayed on the wall.

The large reception desk faced a corridor of seats where the patients sat. I settled myself beside Mum and helped myself to a glossy magazine. I was fascinated by Hugh Grant's resolve to lead a celibate life when the receptionist interrupted. 'Are you Nicola?'

'Yes,' I said.

'I'm sorry about the wait. Would you like some coffee?'

'No.' Mum nudged me. 'Thank you,' I added.

A large jabbering man in his fifties lumbered past me. I'm sure he was going to the heart place, but he walked straight past it and kept walking to the dentist.

'I can't find your appointment card,' said the flustered receptionist. 'I'm going to have a nervous breakdown'.

'Well, you're in the right place for it,' said Mum. And I laughed.

The receptionist gave a titter and kept inspecting her cards.

At that moment, a lean, attractive man with hairy tanned legs jogged up the stairs. He had a Walkman on. *He probably combs his legs,* I thought. He jogged into the heart place.

A boy emerged from behind a dark-blue door. 'See you next time, Paul,' called a deep, crunchy voice. Paul walked carefully out to the dentist, where he must have realized he was going the wrong way because he turned back towards the exit door and kept walking.

So seeing a psychiatrist has that effect on people, I thought.

'Nicola?' said a large man with spiky hair.

'Yes?' I said.

'Come this way.'

I walked into the narrow blue room. Taking in the stacks of files at the back of the room, I searched for the long black couch like in the movies. Instead, two grey chairs sat bleakly beside a desk. Against the desk leaned a white shopping bag with 'Mental Health Convention, Los Angeles 1992' printed in red. It gaped slightly, so I quickly peered into it to see a Nike shoe.

He shook my hand. I expected a firm grip. Instead a wet-fish handshake greeted me.

He said, 'Have a seat.' I knew I'd better be careful with my behaviour from here on.

Which chair shall I take? I wondered. *The one next to the door or the one near the desk?* The one near the door may mean that I want to escape, so I took the one next to the desk.

'So you're Nicola' interrupted my thoughts. 'Did you bring the letter from your doctor? . . . Yes, well, I see you are having a few problems.'

Should I hold my hands or let them flop? I wondered. 'Mmmm . . .' I answered.

The interrogation began.

- 'Who is in your family?'
- 'Who is the boss in your family?'
- 'Have you always lived in the same house?'
- 'How do you get on with your father?'
- 'Does your sister get on with your mother?'
- 'Is the cat an important family member?'
- 'What school do you go to?'

He was peering at my bogey green jumper. The whole time he asked me questions, his hand went like a bullet—jot, jot, jot. Suddenly he clasped his mouth shut. *Achoo! Achoo! Achoo!* He rummaged in his desk drawer and came out with a nasal spray. Two quick squirts later, he was back to it.

- 'Tell me about your friends and boyfriends?'
- 'Why did you break up with your boyfriend?'
- 'Did you use protection?'

I couldn't believe he asked me these things.

- 'Do you have sleeping problems? . . . What, up until 4 a.m.? How long has this been going on for? . . . Really! Sixteen months.'

'Anybody else in your family? It says in this letter that you have been uncooperative, refusing to go to school, lying in bed all day, and angry all the time.'

'I s'pose so,' I mumbled hunched over.

'Sit up straight and look at me,' said Dr D.

Wow, he was a teacher as well! He looked at me. 'Now what would you like to say about it?'

I looked away from his steady stare. But wait, was this a game of who looks away first?

I stared back at him hard as I listed my complaints. 'I feel grouchy all the time. I get so worked up at night I can't sleep. I cry for no reason, and if I'm looking forward to something, I must pull out at the last minute because a feeling takes over me. I'm controlled by my moods, and I try hard to fight them, act normal. I get told to pull it together and not to be lazy. One person offered an exorcism.' My words tumbled out, in a hurry to have my say. I was crying by this time. But it was a comfortable cry. Like things would be taken care of or everything would be all right.

'Well, Nicola, I have good news. There is a lot we can do to help you and you can do to help yourself. Just think of these sessions as skills for life.' I relaxed and listened to what he had to say.

CHAPTER 7

More Chaos

We saw the private psychiatrist about fifteen times. The Prozac at 20 mg produced all the serotonergic side effects—nausea, dizziness, headache, and lethargy—so it was reduced to 5 mg and then 2.5 mg, and we received the following notes:

> August 1995
>
> There is still that slightly precocious, intrusive, mildly out-of-control quality to her, and she is certainly very dominating of her (at one level) rather unassertive parents.
>
> September 1995
>
> Even on the small dose of Prozac, she was getting mood instability effects with periods of hypomania with five days of continuously overly exuberant, socializing, elated mood, overtalkative, not sleeping, mind racing, feeling very distractible, and she has gradually come out of these. She still has times of low mood, and some of these

would come on quite intensely and unexpectedly within a day. She also describes symptoms like anxiety attacks, also associated with depressive feelings of hopelessness. At times she has rages, which she takes out on her mother. She has threatened suicide several times—in fact many times—but has never really acted out on this. We will continue Clonazepam prn at night and a low dose of Melleril to ensure a good sleep pattern, and if further depressive symptoms emerge, then Doxepin in low dose. If she tends to get antidepressant-induced hypomania, then we should be cautious with antidepressants. She may have a predisposition to have a mood disorder of a bipolar type, and these might be the early prodromal signs.

October 1995

It has become clear that the last sixteen months has been very disturbing in terms of her attendance at school. She gets frustrated at her inability to get to sleep and has rages. There is an extremely significant family history of mood disorder with two suicides. There is an indication for a trial of Lithium 750 mg and Melleril 70 mg.

December 1995

At home, things continued to deteriorate over the next year, with rages occurring every day. It was not uncommon for her to rip posters from her bedroom wall, throw items everywhere, and hurl hostile comments at everybody. I was uneasy about leaving her at home; yet if I took her on errands, it would end with us in a shouting match, her jumping from the moving car, or screaming abuse at me on the footpath. I would ring the psychiatrist occasionally for advice. His technique would be to go silent for long periods, and I never knew if he was just thinking, or it was some technique for me to solve my own problems. Inevitably a bill would arrive . . . Sixty dollars for the phone call comprised of mainly silence.

About this time, Nicola said that she could see an angel on the ceiling, and this meant she had to die. I knew that she was keeping knives in her room, and we reported this at the next session, only for me to be told that kids are always threatening to 'top themselves'. I felt disturbed by his callous phrase and felt very uneasy about having any more contact with him for the time being.

All this time, Nicola was getting increasingly irritable and saying she had electric shocks going through her head. Another strange occurrence was her saying that she couldn't walk, but at other times, her legs would work perfectly. It was thirty years before we found out the reason for this.

At the times she would feel physically immobilized, she said she also felt like she wanted to die. Some Lithium carbonate was prescribed for her, which at 0.7 mmols/L was at an ideal serum level. This appeared to help the high feeling, but then clumps of hair appeared in the shower. The first few weeks that her hair started to fall out, she quickly gained weight.

The doctor still remained convinced that it was a parenting problem. I started to question myself and wished I had a video to show what was going on.

CHAPTER 8

A Mixed State

I learnt to keep my distance from Nicola if she was thwarted in any way, as trouble could escalate very quickly. Initially it seemed when Nicola was focussing on her hair at age eleven, that it was a problem of anxiety or panic. However, that was soon to be replaced by stronger emotions such as rage or agitation. She could flip from depression and feeling worthless to giddy conversations on the phone, all the while having tremendous problems falling asleep before 4 a.m. At one stage her sleeping pattern was completely reversed, sleeping 8 a.m. to 5 p.m. She said she dreaded consciousness and would rather be dead. All I could think to do with the insomnia was to use up some cortisol. We often walked the streets starting at 11 p.m. when it would be clear that there would be no sleep that night. At other times she would oversleep, and once, she slept in bed for four days straight. Her biological clock was completely unhinged.

Feeling tired and wired at the same time led her to do destructive things in a desperate attempt to find some relief. She would throw objects, hit out at people, and slam her fist against the car door or make holes in the wall. Sometimes, in a rage, she would rip posters off the wall. She refused to put her seat belt on, always praying for a car accident so that she would be killed. She wished that there would be such a big earthquake she would die. Her favourite spot was on any bridge, as she was convinced that this would be the first to collapse in an earthquake. She tried to cut her arms but could get no further than a scratch as it hurt too much, she said. Her moods were totally unstable. Depression could be there in the morning, and she could be talking suicide; but by evening she would be calling her friends, working her way through every friend in her notebook, in real party mode.

I believe that she deteriorated terribly after being given an antidepressant for depression early on in her treatment. Instead of alternating between highs and lows, she developed a mixed mood. A few years later she was given steroids for sinus, asthma, and ulcerative colitis. Even if she had a mood stabilizer to counter the effect (as some doctors claimed that it would), her mood worsened, and she had to spend some time in hospital. When she originally started showing signs of mania, she maintained that she could read a Bible by running her hands over the pages and could see angels on her bedroom ceiling. She also declared that I was adding poison to her meals and, more bizarrely, that her arms had been burnt by the microwave. She could feel her teeth getting bigger and smaller in her mouth and sense electric shocks in her head.

It was always difficult to know if the anxiety component was a symptom of a mixed state or if it was a separate condition. Even today it is still not confirmed, but she has the 'honour' of being the most anxious person one psychiatrist had ever seen.

These mixed states can become very noisy. Nicola's voice became very voluble, and she came across as demanding and extremely intimidating, stubborn, sarcastic, and an expert at starting arguments. Everything was urgent to her, and she would shout to get her point across. I would be scuttling around closing windows to muffle her noise, and removing anything that could be thrown, always trying to distract her rather than meet her demands. When nothing was working, I would bundle her into my car, any time of the day or night and drive around the suburbs hoping that her shouting could not be heard through the glass windows. She had plenty to say about my driving standards, and of course was completely oblivious to her own disruption to the driver. She would think nothing of winding down the window and shouting profanities to pedestrians. If I could drive around to about 4 a.m. there was a good chance that she would doze. All the time I would be wondering if I should drive this crazed person to the hospital or the police station. One tactic I used when driving her was to look out the driver's side window, being careful not to catch her eye in case she accused me of observing her, which could lead to a confrontation. I continued to be offended by the comment that Nicola just had a behaviour problem and wished that I had a video to show what was going on. I wondered if I was imagining this as mental illness or she was playing to the gallery. I needed to document a couple of days to get this straight in my mind.

CHAPTER 9

Two Days in the Life of Nicola

Tuesday, 14 May 1996

7:30 a.m.

(Practicing our new techniques suggested by Dr D.)

'Nicola, get up.'

'Nicola, it's time to get up.' (shouted, no response, pulled the curtain, shook her)

'F— off, I'm not getting up.'

'Yes, you are. Get out of bed now, or I will pull out you.'

(R. pulled her foot)

'Don't you touch me. Touch me one more time and I'll get you.'

(R. pulled her foot.)

'Okay, okay. I'm getting up.'

'It surprised me to hear Dad's voice. My ears wanted to block out the noise.'

8:30 a.m.

'Mum, can you take me to school?'

'Yes, but all those piercings. You know they are banned.'

'I know, but nobody will notice. Just eyebrow and lip ring.'

'Sounds like wishful thinking to me. I'll expect a phone call from the school within ten minutes'.

'Whatever! I need to go now, before the bell rings'.

9:05 a.m.

I made a phone call to the school office asking for the Dean to call me back, which he did ten minutes later. I told him that Nicola's mood was unstable, and I was worried that she would cause a scene about the piercings.

3:30 p.m.

'I see you have still got your piercings in.'

'Yeah, Tamara had to go to the Dean's Office and saw a note "To All Staff" which said "Please do not comment on Nicola P's piercings. This will be dealt with by the Guidance Counsellor".

I was so impressed at the way this incident was handled by staff in this enormous high school. They took time to deal with a situation that could have easily turned into an ugly showdown.

7:30 p.m.

Nicola started groaning noises and complained that she had a temperature. She then panicked about 'bad thoughts'. I gave her four suggestions. When she continued, I shouted at her to stop and left the house for thirty minutes. When I came home, she was quietly doing her homework.

10:00 p.m.

Nicola was in bed when she called out that she could see faces. She asked me to sleep with her. After lying down on her bed, she started getting abusive, so I left. After twenty minutes she came to my room and apologized and chatted for a bit and went back to her own bed.

Wednesday, 15 May 1996

7:00 a.m.

Nicola wouldn't get up. I pulled off her blankets and yelled, 'If you don't get up in sixty seconds, there will be severe consequences.' I pulled her feet off the bed, and she got up finally.

7:10 a.m.

Laughing while eating breakfast.

7:50 a.m.

>Nicola declares that she is sick, followed by a stream of swearing, mostly about me being a bitch.

8:00 a.m.

>Nicola got into the car and apologized to me for swearing.

3:00 p.m.

>I picked her up to go to the GP. On the way, Nicola bashed the side of the car door and said she had AIDS. I ignored her, and a rage started. She lashed out at me and screamed out that she was not a hypochondriac and that I was mocking her.

3:20 p.m.

>She just stood still on the pavement and would not go into the doctor's building. I told her we were late for the appointment. She didn't move, and I shouted at her to walk. Nicola said she was getting back in the car and not going to a doctor. She raged in the car on the way home. I said, 'I feel like filming you so that Dr D. can see your behaviour.' On reaching the house, I asked her to do her dishes left out on the bench. She protested slightly but did them.

12:30 a.m.

>After lying in bed two hours, she had a panic attack, couldn't breathe, and was furious that she couldn't sleep. Nicola announced that she had silly thoughts and wanted to die. I sat with her for a while waiting

for her to calm herself down. After thirty minutes, she vaulted out of bed, down the hall, and out into the street in her pyjamas. She yelled to me, 'I'm going to kill myself'. I followed her down the road in the car and convinced her to get back in the car. She complied but said, 'You can't stop me killing myself. I've hidden plenty of knives, you f—en bitch.'

The next morning, after a sleepless night, I rang the psychiatrist to have the usual one-way conversation and to receive no help.

CHAPTER 10

Second Opinion

After fifteen sessions with the first psychiatrist and seeing no progress, we decided to move on to get a second opinion. At this time Nicola was starting to take an interest in anything related to the Christian religion. She joined two churches, one traditional and the other Pentecostal. The Pentecostal church offered a free but untrained counsellor, and Nicola latched on to this kind woman who tried to set her on a straight path. Previously the only reference Nicola had made to religion was when she saw angels on the ceiling when she was lying in bed during a depressed stint. Nicola got the good advice to always keep taking her medication, which I was relieved about, so I offered to drive her to this huge church every week. I also relished the respite of an hour.

When she was nearly sixteen, I went ahead with the second opinion. For this Nicola required a referral from her GP. The referral listed her previous medications as Prozac, Lithium, Melleril, Clonazepam, Temazepam, and finished by saying the earlier psychiatrist felt that it was not a bipolar disorder but a personality or behavioural disorder.

Nicola was to continue her behaviour modification (parents pulling her out of bed), and the sleep strategies learnt from the clinical psychologist. The referral was to a child and adolescent psychiatrist. I had mistakenly thought that was what the first psychiatrist was and was concerned that he had led me to believe he had the training to deal with this situation.

I thought that the best way to make a fresh start was to get my point of view across early and ask Nicola to write down hers before the next assessment. I also included a diary of Nicola's typical behaviour over a few days. A year had now passed since Nicola's initial appointment with the first psychiatrist. I wrote out my thoughts.

10 May 1996

She has overwhelming mood swings which happen at any time. The moods are powerful and disruptive and not planned. They can come at time when she has been looking forward to something. She is totally immobilized by them, and each one is destroying her self-esteem. They can happen in public, with friends and family, and do not appear to be linked to any triggers. They can last for hours, during which time her thoughts are irrational and illogical. She has never before had behaviour problems. It started at intermediate school with small panic attacks, which led to rages and not being able to sleep. She has been taught to take control of the moods by grounding, relaxation, exercise, affirmations. They helped a lot at normal times but were ineffective when a mood was there. The moods are totally disabling, and she is no longer able to carry on with schoolwork and relationships with friends. She is unable to attend school more than 30 per cent of the time. Behaviour modification is of no consequence to prevent or curtail a mood in full swing. Methods of hypnosis work well at normal times, and she realizes how low her self-esteem is. She feels so bad when, in a rage, she wants to kill herself. It would be easier than constantly fighting off the moods, she says.

> She has struggled with this problem for two years and is fully aware of the disruption to her life and sees hope for the future if this problem can be brought under control. She has lost concentration and motivation. She feels guilt and disbelief afterwards at the rages. They have become worse in the last week, with a violent rage most days. She has complained of strange thoughts that frighten her.

Nicola also wrote some comments from her perspective.

> I hate getting high. I can be obnoxious and blurt out my problems, exaggerating them, not for sympathy but because I get so passionate with them. The greatest thing is that I believe in God and spend a lot of time with her. I pray to her all the time for normal feelings, and she blessed me with Clonazepam. But I can only stay on it for three months, and I am praying for a long-term drug.

CHAPTER 11

Some Headway

We were impressed with an immediate appointment for the second opinion. The private male psychiatrist led us to a small room, and after a history was taken, I was asked to leave the room for a while so he could speak privately with Nicola. I gathered it was to ask about abuse. After about an hour, he proffered a diagnosis of bipolar affective disorder and offered to send a copy of his notes to the first psychiatrist. After a week of digesting this diagnosis, I made another appointment with him, who was livid. He said that I had 'led the second psychiatrist up the garden path'.

This was the report from the second psychiatrist:

> Certainly Nicola feels that these mood swings are 'ruining' her life, whatever the aetiology, and maybe whatever the aetiology, these should be addressed in a specialist in-patient facility, depending on what you think, as I think a completed suicide attempt is a possibility, not so much right now, but in the medium-term future if she loses hope or does not improve symptomatically. It is possible that she does not suffer a bipolar disorder and these symptoms are due to

psychosocial factors entirely. It is very important that we work together as a team of course, and that I do not encourage any 'splitting'.

He added that it made sense to enrol Nicola with the public health system and that he also worked there and could see Nicola there. He said that he was familiar with a doctor from a specialist child and adolescent hospital who dealt with similar cases.

Over the next few months, Nicola's behaviour became increasingly disturbing. She was convinced that her father and I were the enemy and that she needed to live elsewhere. One night at midnight, she set off walking down the road to find somewhere else to live. She could not even be convinced to wait until daylight. At this point I felt so defeated I went back to bed. I felt so burnt out with trying to reason with her that for the next hour I felt numb. Now, of course, I realize that if I had been thinking more clearly, I could have rung the police and told them a mentally ill fifteen-year-old girl was wandering the streets looking for somewhere to live.

I got a phone call an hour later. It was my parents chastising me after Nicola had arrived on their doorstep. In their view, I needed to take more control. All very well when they had no idea of the situation and no interest in learning more about it. The following day I dropped them a leaflet explaining mood disorders. I doubt that it was read, as the subject was never brought up again.

One morning she decided to sit in the middle of the road in her pyjamas, but her reason for doing so was vague. Luckily, we lived in a no exit street so that there was no traffic. I was totally bewildered by this behaviour and so was a neighbour who berated me about it. Even though this neighbour knew something was amiss, it was once again another judgement on my parenting style.

I kept the staff at high school informed, and they were amazingly supportive, discreet, and surprisingly knowledgeable. They were fully prepared to make allowances for her odd behaviour. Unbelievably, they also decided to allow her to break the rules and allow her piercings. Another student told me she had seen a note to teachers which said they were to make no comment on her piercings or behaviour. The many allowances for her continued for which I was grateful. I had continuous problems wrangling her into her uniform and into the car. Inevitably, she would be very late to class and would stand up on a chair and be disruptive with a loud voice until a friend would tell her to sit down and pipe down.

Was there no part of her life that this disorder did not infiltrate?

CHAPTER 12

An Evening Walk

It was 11 p.m., and I could hear some quiet pacing in the next room. The footsteps became more frenzied, and five minutes later, I heard the clunk of shoes being hurled again and again at the bedroom wall. The sounds resonated through the house, and I thought of how this was becoming a predictable pattern. Each night, Nicola's agitated energy built, and I needed to act swiftly to avoid a massive disturbance to the household and the neighbourhood. Grabbing my slippers, I burst into her bedroom and unearthed her dressing gown from a pile of discarded clothing.

'Time to walk!' I barked as I flung her dressing gown to her. As Nicola grappled with the sleeves and knotted the belt, I was already steering her out of the house, down the driveway, and to the footpath. From here we marched briskly downhill. Occasionally, she put her arm through mine then flinched and whipped it away. For ten minutes, we trekked down the street, crossed over the road, and walked up the other side. We were puffing a little as we maintained the pace. As we walked, I marvelled at the stillness of the street. Occasionally there would be a light playing through the trees, and apart from some leaves rustling, certainly no other sounds. Each house we passed was silent. No shouting, screaming, shrieking. Nicola gripped and released my arm, mute, her face set. What a weird sight we were. Two ghostly figures in flapping dressing gowns on some mission. After a twenty-minute walk, and as we returned to the house, I felt my stomach muscles start to tighten. Adrenaline coursed through me, and it crept down my arms so that my fingernails were now tingling. This was the start to another long night. I ordered myself to calm down. I knew the routine. The minute we returned home, Nicola would fling herself on her bed, and within minutes, there would be a request bellowed at me.

'Mum, do something to my legs. They are killing me'.

That something involved me kneading her calf muscles to quell the restlessness and dampen the shooting pains. At an appointment weeks later, I learned that this muscle tension can be caused by various drugs; and in Nicola's case, it was the typical antipsychotic called Haloperidol. It had a name, akathisia, and this gives a feeling of inner restlessness and the urge to move. While it could be crossing and uncrossing legs, it could be rocking or lifting feet as if marching. It is diagnosed in only 26 per cent of patients. I could imagine that if it is not diagnosed, it could be a reason to stop taking the medication. It is usually grouped with extrapyramidal symptoms which could later turn into tardive dyskinesia, a horrible and almost permanent movement disorder. When it was mentioned to the doctor, he said there were some solutions. Two of them were to change to a modern antipsychotic or to add Cogentin to your mix of medications. Unfortunately, Cogentin has its own side effects, namely a dry mouth and blurred vision among others. For Nicola, this necessitated a visit to the Two-Dollar Shop to find some glasses with the strongest magnification and to set up a row of water bottles by her bed. From then on, Nicola always carried a water bottle and constantly sipped on it throughout the day.

CHAPTER 13

Stigma

Stigma refers to a cluster of negative attitudes and beliefs that motivate the general public to fear, reject, avoid and discriminate against people with mental illness.

In psychiatry there is a system for classifying patient's problems, and it is likely that different doctors seeing the same person with the same description of their problems will not reach the same conclusion about their classification. Reliability when it comes to psychiatric diagnoses seems to be very poor, as it relies on the psychiatrist's snapshot judgement, especially for an initial interview. The classification you get can be more to do with the doctor's preconception than what the actual problems are. A depressed woman who has tried to be well presented with clean hair and make-up is immediately at a disadvantage for a wrong diagnosis. She is assumed to be too functional to be sick. Nobody inquires as to who is in the background washing her clothes or waking her up to get to the appointment. A stressed and anxious person, stating they wish they could end it all may present as a personality disorder, as had happened to Nicola. To make it worse, an initial diagnosis once given is often not discarded; rather, new ones can be added, with all the consequences this may bring.

The *DSM-5* (2013) is the diagnostic tool most widely used by mental health professionals and follows a multiaxial system with five separate axes of diagnosis. Axis I disorder refers to all psychological disorders except mental retardation and personality disorders. It includes anxiety, dissociative, eating, mood, sexual, sleep, psychotic, somatoform, and substance-related disorders. Axis II disorder refers to mental retardation and personality disorders such as antisocial, borderline, and paranoid disorders. The separation of Axis I and Axis II disorders has an impact on several factors, including life course, clinician's willingness to treat, treatment options, and prognosis, all of which interact to influence the amount of stigma associated with each type of disorder.

Axis I disorders are generally seen as treatable and tend to have a shorter life course than Axis II disorders. The Axis II disorders are usually thought of as being chronic or lifelong, some of which may fade out at around age forty. Clinicians are usually open to treat a variety of patients with Axis I clinical disorders such as depression, anxiety, schizophrenia, and specific phobias; however, they are reluctant to treat patients with Axis II disorders due to the stigma of being very difficult to treat. This then creates new barriers to receiving treatment. The differential stigma experienced by patients with an Axis II disorder in the form of less treatment availability is undeniable, and it affects all subsequent interactions in which their deviant label becomes a self-fulfilling prophecy they cannot escape from.

The first time that Nicola was admitted to the ward, she received a classification on Axis II as *Cluster B*, which includes such personality disorders as antisocial, borderline, histrionic, and narcissistic. These disorders are characterized by dramatic, overly emotional, or unpredictable thinking or behaviour. It does not take much to receive a label, which is then ingrained forever in future reports. As it can take at least an hour to carry out a full assessment of a personality disorder, I believe that unless this is specially requested or the client is fortunate enough to have a conscientious clinician, it is not done.

Nicola received her Cluster B label on the first day of her initial admittance to the ward. She noticed that her three orange tablets of Carbamazepine were missing from the paper cup handed to her by her nurse. When querying this, the nurse said the consultant had asked for these to be removed. Nicola immediately panicked, as she relied on these to get to sleep at night. She saw the consultant in the ward office and tapped on the window to get his attention. He was typing and looked up, and Nicola mouthed to him, 'Where is my Carbamazepine?'

'That's it. No more will be given to you,' he answered, and he resumed typing.

'My doctor put me on this, and it is so great. I get heaps of sleep on this, and I never want to come off it. Please, ring my doctor and check with him.'

The consultant shook his head and focussed on his typing. By now Nicola was shouting and pounding on the glass window.

'If I can't have this, then I am walking out of here now. It's the only way that I can get to sleep. Nothing else works.'

'Okay, I will take that into consideration and ring him.'

That phone call took forever. Ten minutes of an intense discussion ensued, with Nicola trying to decipher his body language. At last he looked at her and informed her that the Carbamazepine was to be reinstated. She thanked him and left to find the nurse.

From that time on, Cluster B traits appeared in every report, and it was to cause much consternation to Nicola. This one event was to colour every interaction with staff and was the commencement of a decade of judgement and discrimination as staff took on board this label.

CHAPTER 14

Plagued by Diagnosis

I tried to attend every appointment with Nicola, but I missed one appointment with a male nurse. Nicola reported to me that the nurse had been particularly aggressive and demanded to know why she hadn't been for an interview to work at the Warehouse. I was appalled at this inappropriate suggestion. This was a real setback for Nicola, who had only started to get some confidence to attend appointments on her own. Also, she was still very unwell and could not be an advocate for herself. Obviously, this nurse had got no further than reading Cluster B on Axis II and had decided a huge shakeup was in order for this malingerer. Nicola repeated his comments over and over for the next week when she couldn't sleep. I was extremely annoyed by the damage he had done; and when I asked to meet with him, he refused, saying he felt 'unsafe.' I was amused by this, as I had read in a psychiatrist's notes that I, the mother, was 'demure'.

One time, after Nicola presented at ED for bad akathisia (restlessness in muscles), the registrar, after glancing at the computer record, immediately inquired if she 'felt empty inside' or had 'been cutting' or 'been sexually abused'?

Another psychiatrist insisted that she pull up her sleeves so he could examine her arms for cutting. Another noticed a scratch on her arm and didn't believe her when she said it was from her frisky cat. Another nurse would roll her eyes at another nurse whenever Nicola approached. These comments were very puzzling, but it was not until I saw a discharge sheet that it all fell into place.

Discharge DSM-IV

1. Bipolar disorder NOS
2. Cluster B personality traits
3. Ulcerative colitis, in good control
4. Limited social support, isolation

This diagnosis plagued her everywhere and became a self-fulfilling prophecy from which Nicola could not escape. Whenever Nicola was struggling and called the crisis team, the response was always to 'have a Milo, a bath, call your nurse next week', or one of the worst illogical responses, 'You are on a truckload of medication. There is nothing we can do.'

They gave Nicola the impression that she was exasperating, deviant, difficult, and wasting their time, when all she wanted was to be taken seriously. This Cluster B classification seemed to overshadow the classification of bipolar and its treatment until an overseas-trained psychiatrist challenged the diagnosis, which made a massive difference for future treatment. The Axis II diagnosis changed from Cluster B to Personality NOS (not otherwise specified).

It is possible that the poorer prognosis associated with Axis II personality disorder is because of the limited treatment options available and reflects a research bias and, hence, a lack of interest from pharmaceutical companies. Whatever, the stigma resulting in fewer treatment methods and access experienced by patients with an Axis II disorder is undeniable.

Aside from the negative effects of labelling from clinicians, our culture promulgates negative views of mental illness. The general understanding of mental illness comes from distorted and exaggerated portrayals rather than from everyday encounters. We hear terms such as *crazy*, *insane*, *psycho* and *mental*. In addition, the media often portray mentally ill people as those who commit violence; however, studies show that those with mental health disorders are no more likely to commit violent crimes than people in the general population. There is also a general stigma associated with mental illness that shows in our social media. There are alerts put out on Neighbourly, a forum where neighbours can chat in New Zealand, which often insinuates that oddly dressed or wandering people should 'be reported' as they may be dangerous. This is especially so that now many properties have cameras set up to catch such occurrences. It can happen that ten or twelve contributors will all exercise their imagination and add their scary stories and judgments. They incorrectly assume that these stragglers are not trying hard enough or don't want to get better. The belief is that if you're struggling with mental health, a competent therapist and a pill or two can easily remedy the situation. This social ostracism criticizes the patient and the already overburdened families.

After twenty-six years of seeing various clinicians, a locum threw a wrench in the works for Nicola. By now she had confidently been given the bipolar diagnosis, and it seemed we were on the right track. Not so.

Apparently, Nicola had made a comment that she felt so bad she felt like dying or wanted to kill herself. It was a throwaway comment, and rather than investigating further, this clinician changed her diagnosis back to borderline with cyclothymia. We were back to square one again. We challenged this new diagnosis with her next clinician, who got very defensive on behalf of the locum and huffily announced that he and the locum had trained at the same institute in London and knew what they were talking about. It is nearly impossible to challenge a psychiatrist, as the profession is still dominated by clinicians who hold a lot of privilege.

This negative image needs to change. Someday, perhaps, we'll be as accepting when talking about people with mental health disorders as we are today when talking about people with cancer or heart disease.

CHAPTER 15

Post-Traumatic Stress Disorder (PTSD)

We all hope to have a brain that is working at an optimal level. What can get in the way is stress. There are two types of stress, normal and extreme. Normal stress usually resolves in a few minutes, whereas extreme stress can leave you trapped in a survival mode for years.

Dr J. Ford and J. Wortman (2013) explain that we first need to learn that there are three basic levels of the brain. For your brain to operate at an optimal level, we need the first level, the reptile brain (amygdala), which ensures the body receives enough oxygen, food, and liquids to stay alive. It works automatically like a robot. It is not designed to keep us from danger, only to keep our basic bodily functions intact.

The second level, the palaeomammalian (the emotional brain) includes the alarm, reward centre, and several other nearby areas that enable us to feel basic emotions such as fear, anger, satisfaction, and happiness. This alarm teams up with the reptile brain to keep us alive, as well as getting us to pay attention to pleasure. When they function well, life is fulfilling. When they work at cross-purposes, the emotional brain can cause us a great deal of stress. For instance, the reward centre may demand that we go skydiving, while the alarm screams that it is not safe to jump out of a plane.

Thankfully, we have a third level of the brain, the learning, thinking, or non-mammalian brain. It is the command centre and the decision-maker. It catches and filters the messages from the alarm and reward centres by using the brain's memory centre. The memory centre screens messages without judgment, looking for those that are familiar. The main problem for the three team members is that the alarm and reward centres can become so demanding that they can overwhelm the memory centre. (By the way, it is the alarm brain that communicates with the reptile brain and gives orders to speed up or slow down our heart or breathing rate.)

As thinking is our brain's greatest power, our ability to use it is our greatest opportunity to reduce stress.

Most of the time, the alarm brain is helpful, like when it alerts you that your pot is boiling over. This alarm, with a little surge of adrenaline, can give you a gentle nudge to act. The problem is when the alarm misfires. This happens when the brain's alarm can't tell the difference between a survival threat and an ordinary event—for example, when a car backfiring sounds like a gun. When stress causes our brain to misread situations, it can lead to overreactions because the brain's alarm becomes overly sensitive. If we don't recognize the onset of extreme stress until it is too late, we feel overwhelmed and ready to explode. Most of us don't know how to turn our brain's alarm down when it is stuck in the 'on' position. When the emergency is over, we still react with the same intensity. It doesn't always have to be a trauma of a catastrophic proportion; it could be many small incidents, and it is worse if this trauma happens in childhood or adolescence.

Nicola became ill with anxiety, panic, and prodromal symptoms of bipolar I when she was about twelve years old. By fourteen years, she was showing extreme bipolar I symptoms which were not entirely confirmed until she was an inpatient at a specialist children and adolescent hospital on her sixteenth birthday. Up until then, she had already seen numerous GPs, clinical psychologists, psychotherapists and psychiatrists who, once they had listened to her concerns, mostly downplayed her symptoms as teenage behaviour. One person took it seriously, and that was when she was admitted to this hospital. Unfortunately, former reactions from previous staff included yelling at her, sarcasm, reprimands, lectures, and dressing-downs. As she got older, as well as having to contend with her chaotic mood swings, she had to contend with medications withheld when it was trendy to be on monotherapy, never having any effective medications, scoffing from family members, thousands of nights not being able to sleep, making plans with friends and not being able to follow through, abuse from other patients in the ward, indifferent nurses, and endless anxiety about appointments. She was either agitated and angry, or exhausted and paralyzed in bed—in other words, fight or freeze, both components of PTSD. Trauma may be simply summed up as any negative event that occurs in a state of relative helplessness.

Trauma and most of its effects are recognized in medical care, and sometimes an effort is made to lessen the impact. When she was sixteen, Nicola's psychiatrist tried to avoid her being in an adult ward and exposed to the activity there. At this time adolescent wards were opening, and she was fortunate to be referred to one.

There is a lack of awareness about how traumatizing it can be to live day in and day out with a life-threatening illness. To keep looking for help from medical professionals who can be judgmental and dismissive can also be a source of trauma. If your symptoms aren't responding well to treatment and you have been shamed, perceived as though you were just 'wanting attention', or told you weren't trying, then eventually getting a diagnosis of trauma can be empowering.

CHAPTER 16

You Can Heal and Recover from the Effects of Trauma

In 2019 Nicola came across a book called *Hijacked by Your Brain* by Dr Julian Ford, who introduces an intervention to interrupt and calm alarm reactions. This enabled Nicola to use the thinking parts of the brain, the prefrontal cortex and hippocampus, to focus on an experience that was important to her rather than being driven by problem messages from the amygdala. This shift in focus took a lot of work. It meant focusing on positive emotions, values, goals, and choices. After a few days of practicing, Nicola was able to turn down her alarm a little, and there was improvement in her anxiety and panic. As she became more adept at managing her alarm, her fatigue lifted (the freeze state of PTSD), and she became more alert.

Over the years, from childhood to the age of thirty-nine, there were to be many years of anxiety-provoking situations. Nicola can rattle off many of the traumatizing comments made to her by staff. Lots have been obliterated by Electroconvulsive therapy ECT from her conscious brain, but they no doubt are still there buried deep in the unconscious memory. Every day as she focuses on making new memories and storing them in her vault, she can reset her alarm when it gets frantic. The actual technique of SOS as described by Dr Julian Ford has specific steps to be followed and seems to surpass all previous attempts by Nicola.

However, a person who is psychologically traumatized is physiologically traumatized too. We cannot be angry without our body being angry too. A traumatized individual is entrapped in an altered state of dysregulated arousal. The traumatic material cannot be processed as it normally is, and the body encodes it as present sensations instead of memories of the past.

Traumatic experiences are not stories with beginnings, plot twists, endings, and a flow of details. They are undigested fragments beyond the reach of language. Trauma, although psychological, is held in the body, and the best course of therapy is to find a somatic therapist.

In the *DSM-5*, released in May 2013, PTSD just got more complex when it added a new symptom domain of negative alterations in mood or cognition. As well, the hyperarousal domain now included self-destructive behaviour, and it added a subtype of dissociation. These changes reflected advances in clinical practice, which takes into consideration what trauma survivors had been saying for decades.

Nicola's symptoms made an impact on even routine activities (such as shopping), turning them into almost unmanageable ordeals. Many times, I would have to leave Nicola in the car while I rushed around the supermarket. She could not help me with the simplest of tasks, and there were many times she was barely able to function at all. Making a bed, emptying a rubbish basket, feeding the cat . . . all were totally beyond her. She just couldn't do it. She wasn't lazy, but thinking through the steps floored her. At the time, it seemed preposterous to me that I was continually failing in setting boundaries with her and tolerating unacceptable behaviour. Later I learned that this only works well with rational people, not those with PTSD.

In vogue at the time was a lightweight somatic therapy called EMDR. Nicola was keen to experience it in the hope that it might help her brain and body to self-regulate.

Eye Movement Desensitization and Reprogramming (EMDR) is a therapy for accessing and integrating memory systems. It consists of exposing the client to feared memories in a structured and caring manner. Unlike other methods, it adds a series of eye movements or other forms of sensory stimulation, such as finger tapping, to the process. Its theory is that side-to-side eye movements will trigger memory-updating systems, because they are genetically related to foraging and looking out for predators and prey. This is probably why rapid eye movement (REM) sleep occurs while our brains are engaging in the consolidation of new memory.

The therapists Nicola approached for some sessions were well trained and eager to get to work. After each session, Nicola proudly ran over with me the two or three issues they worked on that day. Things seemed to be going well, and I was starting to entertain high hopes that perhaps she would, after all, make a steady recovery and be able to lead a more 'normal' life. Suddenly it all went wrong. Within twenty minutes of leaving a session, she started to get a flooding of brand-new memories. Then, the memories she thought had been integrated started reappearing in full force. Later we were to learn that the EMDR was not effective for her because she was still experiencing mixed moods from the bipolar. We had mistakenly thought that had already been resolved. As EMDR was put on hold, a new issue unbelievably appeared. This affected Nicola's breathing and brain function, and it took a concerted effort to resolve.

CHAPTER 17

Obstructive Sleep Apnoea

I had always wondered why Nicola could never accomplish an activity. I am not talking about a bush tramp, a shopping trip, hanging out the washing, or emptying the dishwasher. I mean much simpler stuff—putting a milk bottle in the fridge, hanging up a towel, or closing a wardrobe door. And why did she spend so many hours immobile in bed, not sleeping, not reading, not listening to music, or even Facebooking? She seemed dispirited and totally inanimate.

I made plenty of allowances for her. Once the Clozapine had kicked in for the recommended six months, I thought that she would be all action. Not so. Her Diazepam, a muscle relaxant, was reduced by 1mg a week, down to 25mg a day. Maybe that high amount was making her sluggish, and she would soon liven up. But that didn't happen. I decided to insist that she get out of bed when she woke up each morning. That was when Nicola told me she felt she had been hit over the head every morning with an excruciating headache. She had never felt such severe fatigue. As well, her normal day-to-day anxiety was intensifying and now mingling with obsessive thoughts of disasters such as planes crashing on our house . . . the pharmacist forgetting to make her blister pack . . . the local river flooding with the bridge collapsing.

The circular conversations she wanted to have with me were unbearable. We would get to some decision, and within minutes it was back to her questioning me again about what we had decided. I didn't know if it was ruminating or her memory was crumbling. I wrote the answer down, first in her diary and then in super large letters stuck to the wall. I would direct her to the signs every time the subject came up. I also noticed that she couldn't concentrate, which made it difficult for her to even read the signs. I tried to interest her in watching a few minutes of her favourite TV programs. She could barely sit for twenty seconds.

I was on duty every minute of the day. It was a very demanding time for me as she was becoming increasingly irritable and demanding, with zero tolerance for my perceived blunders. The porridge was too hot, the window was opened too wide, and even the flagpole at the school next door flapped too loudly.

Apart from not being able to think properly, she could not partake in a conversation or even listen to the initial sentence of another person talking. I would often forget and start up a conversation, only to have her shut me down when I was halfway through the first sentence. It was a lonely time, as I was not permitted to talk. She would get clearly rattled if I went out of sight, but then she was exasperated if I came too close to her, scratched my arm, or chewed my apple loudly. It was like the old days of being in a mixed mood.

Then the dizziness started. Lying in her bed, she felt as if she was floating in a boat. Getting out of bed had to be done in stages, and even then, walking was done by holding on to the wall or my shoulder like a blind person. She constantly had a low mood, not to the point of depression, but rather seeing the cup as half-empty and being pessimistic. With so little energy, she would be unmotivated to shower or even work out what clothes to wear and would opt to stay in her nightie all day to the point that it was normal to see her totally unkempt. She started to cancel all her medical and dental appointments. If she was out of bed, she would announce that she needed to sit or lie immediately. Standing was out of her capability. With this hypersomnolence, I noticed a large weight gain. In a day, she would maybe clock up two hundred steps in total. I added up her calories. It seemed to always be about 1,500 calories. That seemed about right if she could increase her activity.

All this time there was the awfulness of night sweats. She could wake drenched after being in bed an hour. Her bed would have to be remade three times over, or if it had been an extra-tiring day, she would abandon her bed and move to the spare room, leaving the clean-up for the morning. Sometimes in the night, she would wake up gasping and choking. She would say that she couldn't breathe. The disrupted sleep made her tired the next day. One night I filmed her sleeping with my phone, and her breathing was very noisy. If she had had a partner, it would have been intolerable.

The headaches were becoming unbearable, almost like a migraine which would last until lunchtime. A visit to the GP resulted in a large dose of 80 mg Propranolol in the morning to deal with these migraines. The Propranolol, a beta-blocker, also assisted in lowering her increased heart rate of 148 beats a minute, and the headaches became more bearable.

I decided to google *noisy breathing* and came across Obstructive Sleep Apnoea. It outlined an exact description of Nicola's symptoms. The article recommended a sleep test in a laboratory to determine the severity of the apnoea. As the muscle tone of the body ordinarily relaxes during sleep and the airway at the throat is composed of walls of soft tissue, which can collapse, it is not surprising that breathing can be obstructed during sleep. This is associated with a reduction in blood oxygen saturation.

A call to the local sleep clinic and a delay of four weeks resulted in a courier delivering testing equipment and a questionnaire. It was easy to understand the instructions, and after a night test of eight hours, the equipment was sent to be analysed.

The following week, our appointment with the sleep psychologist revealed why she had been so tired each morning, but it was also very concerning. The results showed between ten and fifteen apnoeas an hour.

An apnoea is where breathing repeatedly stops for a period and then restarts. Her average apnoea lasted fifty-seven seconds. The lowest oxygen saturation was 86 per cent. Repeated cycles of decreased oxygenation can lead to very serious cardiovascular problems.

The next step was to find a solution. The sleep psychologist recommended a CPAP machine, but further investigation showed it wasn't suitable for those with bipolar, as it can cause mania. An alternative was a Mandibular Advancement Device, which is a mouth guard worn at night to hold the jaw and tongue forward. For this, a dentist made an impression of Nicola's teeth and sent it to Australia for a device to be constructed.

The device fitted perfectly, and Nicola took it home to wear in bed overnight. After practicing wearing it for several hours before bed and with some numbing cream applied where it rubbed her gums, the device became comfortable, and she wore it for the entire eight hours. That first morning, she woke up feeling fabulous. No headache, and she could walk easily for the first time in a year. She was able to experience the deep stage of non-REM sleep (stage 3), which is required for the physically restorative effects of sleep and non-REM (stage 2) with REM, which is associated with mental recovery and maintenance. Her obstructive sleep apnoea was rated as moderate and, therefore, dangerous when driving a car.

It was really a simple solution once it was identified, and other than cleaning it daily and remembering to wear it, it was the best investment ever. The device proved to be quite fragile and could split in two if dropped, which did happen twice. Twice it was sent to Australia to be mended, so an extra one was ordered. It also resulted in a weight loss of 8kg just by her wearing it over time. For people who don't have a partner, it could take much longer to diagnose, as the snoring and gasping would not be so clearly heard. Maybe an advertising program on obstructive sleep apnoea could induce harmony in households and reduce the car accident toll, saving many lives. Unfortunately many patients with recognized and unrecognized obstructive sleep apnoea receive hypnotics or sedatives to treat conditions of sleeping difficulties. Concerns have been expressed that administration of these drugs to people with coexisting sleep apnoea may worsen sleep apnoea.

Although we were thrilled with the device, all was not quite well in the mood department. There was still a way to go yet.

CHAPTER 18

Moving to the Public Mental Health Services and Specialist Hospital

It was with some relief that the second private psychiatrist suggested moving from private psychiatrists to the publicly funded community mental health. It was because of the long public waiting list that we had opted for private treatment before this. Medical insurance did not cover this treatment. In 1996, eighty-five-minute appointments cost $240 and a phone call $60, so it was some reprieve for the chequebook.

At this stage, Nicola was taking Clonazepam and Temazepam. She had stopped 75 mg Prothiaden for sleep from her GP, and Lithium Carbonate and Fluoxetine from her first psychiatrist.

Her first appointment in the public system took place within two months, and after blood tests were checked, Nicola was prescribed Sodium Valproate, which was built up to 1,600 mg daily. In the beginning, it proved to be at a level of 300, just in the therapeutic range of 300–600.

In August 1996, things started to unravel even more at home. There were still sleep problems, but now there was constant raging and talk of demons and devils. One day she smashed up her room and wouldn't stop screaming. I called the crisis team, who visited at home. They said her behaviour was so bad that she presented as someone who was suffering a borderline personality disorder. In the meantime, they arranged for her to be prescribed 5 mg Haloperidol and 1mg Cogentin.

The next day, we needed to attend an appointment at the community mental health building. After a harrowing trip in the car, when Nicola refused to do up her seat belt and constantly tried to open the car door, we reached the building. As I parked the car, Nicola wound the window down and called out some insults to college girls in uniform. In the reception area, Nicola lay on the floor and crawled under some chairs. She then staggered into the appointment room and ran around in circles until she left for the toilet. The doctor and I stared at this bizarre behaviour. In the doctor's report, he wrote, 'She is certainly capable of the most extraordinary behaviour, the likes of which I have never seen in my seven years or so of practice as a psychiatrist!'

He noted that 'At times her mood has been depressed, but this has only been for an hour or two, but the main problem in the last seven days has been attacks of feeling high, with her thoughts racing, and she experiences dramatically angry feelings welling up from inside of herself which erupt and have a very distressing effect on all those around her. It sounds as if her parents feel quite powerless when she is in this state, and it sounds as if there is nothing they can do or say that makes any difference. My overall impression is that Nicola suffers a genuine bipolar disorder, and sometimes she may be in the throes of a mixed state, i.e. of alternating depression and hypomania within the space of twenty-four to forty-eight hours. Certainly, in the last seven days, it seems as if she has been hypomanic but presenting as irritable and hostile instead of as high, which can sometimes happen'.

He thought an inpatient stay at a specialist children and adolescent hospital would be beneficial, so arrangements were made to go to there for an in-depth assessment and treatment program looking at the cognitive behavioural treatment of mood swings as well as experimenting with medication to try to achieve better prophylaxis.

We had previously booked and paid for a two-week trip to Australia at this time and intended to go. The doctor said it was not a good idea, as she could 'go off' in the plane. He prescribed some Thioridazine and Diazepam, and we decided to go ahead with our plans and hope for the best. The weather was stifling, and the bush fires were well underway. I felt embarrassed staying with family and was on tenterhooks the whole time, waiting for the next eruption. Nicola turned sixteen years old the day we got back, and she was given permission to have one glass only of champagne.

Nicola was to have an EEG and CT scan and then go straight to the specialist hospital's child and family unit for 6 to 8 or 10 weeks.

We left at 5 a.m. in a taxi to catch the early flight to Auckland. None of us were speaking as we fretted about what lay ahead. We delivered Nicola for the 9 a.m. appointment, and we checked into a backpacker. No mobile phones then, so the next few weeks involved several trips a day to the unit to get updates from Nicola and staff. There was a school in the ward, and Nicola soon made some friends there. It worked out well having the adolescents all grouped together, and Nicola likened it to boarding school.

CHAPTER 19

At the Specialist Hospital

Medical care is both a science and an art, and it helps to have positive human emotions. They all play a big part in recovery from an illness.

I have witnessed doctors treating patients as just a lump of flesh to be prodded, injected, weighed, measured, and tested. An important part of the healing process is missing.

On the other hand, there are some doctors who can listen to their patients, reassure them, provide confidence in their healing, and value them as partners in the process. Nicola has encountered several practitioners with these fine qualities.

In the months leading up to Nicola's stay at the specialist hospital, her second psychiatrist did his best to find the right combination of medications to treat Nicola. Never really knowing the exact diagnosis, he tried medications that were designed to address mania, depression, and mood instability. Nothing much was helping. He requested admission to the specialist hospital for an in-depth assessment and treatment program. Even to get a confirmed diagnosis would be an immense help, as so far, the prime aetiology was still undecided.

Nicola felt positive about her admission, as she thought the rules and limits would be good for her.

On checking in, she was on a dose of 600 mg of Sodium Valproate. The level eight hours post dose was 341 μmol/L (normal range was 350–700 μmol/L). By now the Lithium had been stopped because of her weight gain, nausea, tremors, and skin problems. The Haloperidol was exchanged for Thioridazine because of akathisia.

A few days before being admitted, Nicola described rubbing her fingers over a book and being able to read words that appeared on her fingers. She accused people in the house of poisoning her food and setting things up so that she would fail. Apart from a later episode concerning birds when her mixed mood was extreme, this was as much psychosis ever to be witnessed in thirty years.

Nicola was able to make friends in the ward, especially with those who seemed to have her symptoms. There was a schoolroom where teachers attempted to get the patients to do some arts and crafts, such as making Christmas cards and posters. It was a little difficult for them, as some of the patients were trying new medications and could only doze on couches.

Nicola's discharge summary noted that although she appeared hypomanic throughout her stay, by her own self-report, was very settled. Probably what partially gave this away was the way she dressed in a very short miniskirt and a top with a bare midriff. She was asked to cover up with a change of clothes. She was noted to be very bouncy and overly familiar. Her speech was mildly pressured with no evidence of a formal thought disorder or psychotic features. The best piece of news was that her diagnosis was confirmed as bipolar disorder not otherwise specified—not a borderline personality disorder. Her bipolar had rapid cycling, depression, and atypical features. There was no mention of mixed mood.

Nicola arrived home in a cheerful mood, with a different regime of medication. She agreed to join an adolescent psychotherapy group.

However, it was not long before she tried to make two unprovoked attacks on me. Also, she began sleeping with knives in her bed and looking for pills to kill herself if I left the house. I think this was caused by a dose of 40 mg Prozac, which elevated her. It was very disappointing.

Although we were very grateful for Nicola's admission to the hospital, it almost seemed that we were back to where we started. Something was still very wrong.

CHAPTER 20

Crazy Mental Health Assistance

This process would test the stamina and perseverance of the most seasoned patient. After a flare of ulcerative colitis, Nicola was losing ground. Night after night of failing to sleep until 7am because of physical and emotional pain was turning her into a fiend with distorted thinking and a prickly exterior. Snatching some sleep from 7 a.m. to 11 a.m. was a major feat. Sleep was number 1 on the list to prevent a relapse into a brute of a mixed mood. Whacking her head and punching the bed, dog-tired with a brain that would not shut down, the long weekend was in sight.

Action needed. Off to an early start. First phone call was Friday 8 a.m. to community mental health. The receptionist rang for Nicola's nurse, and a message was left. The nurse returned the call with the promise to speak to a psychiatrist. Nicola's usual psychiatrist was overseas for three weeks, and there was no locum. After some phone tag, it appeared that there was no doctor at all available that day.

Just a script of Chlorpromazine and Promethazine needed please.

Having waited until 4 p.m., still with the hope of tracking down someone or something to aid sleep, we decided it was time to turn to the usual GP at the medical centre.

Relief as the receptionist answered soon turned to dismay as the receptionist enquired as to what was the reason for requiring an appointment. This seemed to be a triaging receptionist. Confidently, Nicola conveyed to her that she had mental health problems and was asking for a medication for sleep and that this was important, as her mental health was deteriorating with the insomnia.

'Oh no, that is not a reason to come to our after hours. We can't give you an appointment for that kind of thing.'

Nicola got flustered and tried to explain how dangerous it was for her to not be able to sleep and that she had a particular medication prescribed for her before and it sorted her out enough that she could return to normal. Still not convinced, the receptionist firmly shut her down. After another go at explaining, the receptionist passed Nicola to a nurse who expressed her understanding but said that she could not assist as she did not meet the criteria for urgent care.

'Looks like I will have to go to ED and wait six hours to be seen, after the car accidents and sports injuries, or go to after hours in High Street'.

'No,' the nurse said, 'after hours does not accept our patients whilst we are still open.'

Nicola replied, 'But you are open but won't see me, and after hours won't see me because I am a patient at this centre.'

'They will see you when we are not open. That is, after 10 p.m. when we close, and they close at 11 p.m.'

Nicola thought that maybe ED would be better. After all, they do see everyone, especially if you have already tried your own GP. After confirming with a mental health advice line, a decision was made to not go to ED on a Friday night; rather, we would go to after hours on a Saturday, when it allowed those from Nicola's usual medical centre to attend.

CHAPTER 21

Metabolic Monitoring of Antipsychotic Medication

Weight was a topic very much on Nicola's mind. When she was on Lithium, she freaked out when her weight increased from 55 kg to 61 kg. She, being very influenced by peer pressure, saw herself as enormous and insisted that she come off the Lithium. About this time, Thioridazine was discontinued in New Zealand due to possible heart problems it could cause and was replaced with a new atypical antipsychotic named Olanzapine.

All antipsychotics pose a risk of significant weight gain (greater than or equal to 7 per cent of baseline body weight). Olanzapine, Clozapine, and Chlorpromazine are among the worst. Weight became a serious issue for Nicola when she started on Olanzapine. Within a few months, her weight increased to 103 kg, and then it quickly rose to 130 kg.

At this time Nicola thought bariatric surgery was worth investigating—in particular, laparoscopic adjustable gastric banding. We had heard that in the USA, up to 150,000 adult patients undergo bariatric surgery each year. What we didn't know in 1990 was that the alterations made to the gastrointestinal tract in patients who have undergone elective surgery can have a profound impact on drug safety and efficacy.

The absorption of different pharmacologic agents can be drastically altered in these patients. Reducing the size of the stomach can impede the disintegration and dissolution of certain drugs because the gastric mixing is compromised. In some cases, this can be overcome by crushing the tablets or by using a liquid formulation; however, some drugs cannot be crushed or do not come in liquid form.

Restrictive gastric surgeries can often increase gastric pH. The dissolution of acidic or enteric-coated drugs is more likely to be impeded by increases in gastric pH (alkaline is 7–14) as these drugs are more soluble in a lower pH environment. The change in pH causes a decrease in the absorption of any medication that relies on an acidic pH for the absorption of 0–7. Olanzapine requires an acid pH of 2.4. In addition, bariatric surgery can drastically reduce the length and surface area within the GI tract that is available to absorb the drugs.

So at that time, the bariatric lap band sounded like a promising way to keep weight stable. Several clinics had now opened in New Zealand, and Nicola accepted an offer in Auckland to undergo the procedure. This could be the answer to avoid any more weight gain, she thought.

The surgery took place late in the morning, and she was discharged at 5 p.m. She emerged from the recovery room with four tiny scars covered with a sticky plaster and a scar where a port had been placed to inflate the laparoscopic band. Some fluid was put in the band. Nicola thought that it felt tight, and by the next day, she had to return to have some of the fluid extracted.

That was a nuisance, but nothing compared to the evening of the surgery. I noticed Nicola had started to get irritable. She had her usual medication at 7 p.m., and within two hours, she started to get more and more anxious. She wanted to pick a fight with me. I consoled myself by thinking, *Just wait, in twenty-five minutes, her Olanzapine will surely calm her down. It is quick-acting.* But in another two hours, she was lashing out and shouting. Not knowing what to do, I called an ambulance. When they discovered that her dose of Olanzapine was 50 mg, an amount that had been prescribed for her, they monitored her heart. They thought that this was the problem.

Later we were able to look at a chart of poor drug absorption following bariatric surgery. It indicated that Olanzapine, Quetiapine, Metformin, Zolpidem, and Lamotrigine were all drugs whose absorption could be severely impacted by the bariatric surgery. She had been prescribed all these drugs at various times. Eventually, the band needed to be removed and was declared an immense failure. We read later that these weight-loss clinics no longer offered this surgery.

CHAPTER 22

What Is Treatment Resistance in Psychiatry?

Nicola underwent scores of various drug and psychological treatments over the last three decades, none of which ever made a difference to her condition. By about the year 2000, clinicians were starting to mutter about treatment-resistant psychiatric disorders. I wondered whether this definition made sense and what evidence was being used.

In depression, in anxiety disorders, and in schizophrenia, the standard definition is 'an inadequate response to at least two adequate (appropriate dose and lasting for at least six weeks) treatment episodes with different drugs'. A response can be considered inadequate based on an absolute threshold of symptom severity or a percentage change from baseline in symptom severity. In major depression and in generalized anxiety disorder, response is usually defined as a 50 per cent decrease in symptom severity. In obsessive-compulsive disorder, it is usually defined as a 35 per cent decrease in symptom severity.

Response, defined as 'a percentage improvement in the global score of a rating scale', can obscure clinical reality: a response can be seen in a depressed patient despite high residual cognitive symptoms. Functioning or distress are often not considered when defining an adequate response.

It has been suggested that the expression *treatment resistance* is devoid of empathy. The expression seems to blame the disorder or even the patient: a lay press article mentioned that a new antidepressant 'can cause rapid antidepressant effects in many people with "stubborn depression"'.

Finally, the concept of treatment resistance stems from an acute illness model with remission or cure as the goal. Unfortunately, not all patients with psychiatric disorders can reach that symptom-free goal. The use of the more collaborative expression *'difficult to treat' psychiatric disorders* could be preferred, as this may fit better with the recurrent or chronic nature of some psychiatric disorders. Achieving a meaningful life despite limitations can be the goal. This also resonates with the 'recovery' movement, which identifies regaining personal control and establishing a personally meaningful life, with or without residual symptoms, as the objective to pursue.

Over the years Nicola was able to test-drive many drugs and systematically discard all of them. Each drug would be increased in the hope that maybe a higher level may be the answer. Many clinicians were astonished that she could still even walk on the high amounts, but for her it was like taking a sugar pill. Unable to accept the disappointing results, clinicians thought that she was not making an effort, was work-shy, wasting life, being inactive, giving up on friendships, having a bad attitude or even a personality disorder. It became normal for Nicola to be the target of directives to get out of bed and get moving. What they didn't realize was that Nicola was trying to manage while completely unmedicated.

What they were seeing was a person self-isolating due to the severity of the illness. Nicola was fighting, but silently. She was exhausted and too ill to socialize. She cared so much that she was disappointing her support people. One day, fatigued and overwhelmed, she decided that she was too much of a problem and needed to end it all.

She drove herself to the train station, intending to jump in front of a train. When she got there, she found a wire-netting fence lining the railway track. By this time, I realized that the car was missing and phoned the police. They were able to respond, found her, and took her back to the police station. The policewoman had a talk with her, telling her that if she wanted to die, it would be permanent; did she realize this? Nicola looked at her blankly.

This was now a crisis, and I was not able to keep her safe. She had to be admitted to the ward.

Fortunately, this now became the turning point in Nicola's recovery, when she met some incredible advocates, real-life angels.

CHAPTER 23

Rapid Metabolizer

Over the years, as each medication failed to give any relief to Nicola, I could not help but do my own research. I spent hours looking at articles on Google and Google Scholar. I kept coming across how Clozapine could be a miracle drug, especially for those with schizophrenia. Every time I mentioned it to clinicians, I was firmly told that this was not used in New Zealand for bipolar. There was no reasoning for it. It was available but not used in this country. What I couldn't understand was why anyone would deny this option to those patients who didn't want to suffer needlessly.

I managed to get a letter of support for Clozapine from three psychiatrists and a clinical psychologist, which I presented to Nicola's current clinician. The upshot of this was Nicola was prescribed Haloperidol. At very high doses of 35 mg, this did contain her; but once again, she was now criticized for taking an extraordinarily high dose. And of course, there was the danger of the irreversible tardive dyskinesia.

A locum was now involved, who wrote a report diagnosing Nicola as having cyclothymia. I could not believe it. My hopes were dashed. Back to square one.

Shortly after this, I was at breaking point. I contacted crisis resolution services, determined to get this matter settled. I was prepared to go anywhere, even to the media. I was offered an appointment and was much heartened by the report that followed.

Diagnoses:

Axis I: Combined extreme state of agitation and anxiety with reportedly olfactory (odd smells), bodily (felt something is coming out of her body), and auditory hallucinations (sound of birds), with at times paranoid-delusional thinking, anger outbursts, and only partial or insufficient response despite combination of medication and prescription of extremely high doses; warranting diagnosis of probably schizoaffective disorder, bipolar type with significant overlays of anxiety. Neuroleptic-induced akathisia.

Query: High metabolic rate/kindling effect

Axis II: Strong willed and resilient personality traits

Axis III: Ulcerative colitis, well controlled.

Gastric banding removed.

Axis IV: Long-standing mental health issues and related adjustment, having at times become even more complicated in the context of chronic inflammatory bowel disease; understandably struggling despite plethora of psychotropic medication and extremely high doses.

Axis V: GAF: 41

Partnership Plan:

Recommend CT or MRI head, genetic testing for high metabolizing type, ECT continuation, planned voluntary admission to the inpatient unit for further diagnostic clarification and rationalization of medication.

When I saw the partnership plan, I could have been knocked down with a feather. Two words jumped out: *high metabolizing*. At last, some comforting words. Could this be part of the answer even though the report did not include the word *Clozapine*? I needed to investigate this further.

Meanwhile, Nicola became a patient in the ward where she met the psychiatrist who was courageous enough to introduce Clozapine.

By now Nicola was relieved to have her Axis II diagnosis changed, but she was also distraught, thinking nothing would change with her medication. At this point she was taking medication twenty-two times a day.

Morning
Epilim.....................34 mls (liquid)
Tegretol...................24 mls
Microlut..................2
Pentasa....................8 Tabs
Haloperidol..............6 mg
Diazepam.................2.5 mg
Prazosin...................2
Lamotrigine.............50 mg

Noon
Epilim.....................34 mls
Tegretol...................24 mls
Haloperidol..............6 mg

Evening

Epilim	34 mls
Tegretol	24 mls
Prazosin	2
Olanzapine	55 mg
Haloperidol	8.5 mg
Diazepam	5 mg
Solian	300 mg
Lamotrigine	50 mg
Kemadrin	prn

A plan was hatched whereby Nicola's medication was to be rationalized, and Clozapine would be eventually introduced. Nicola was bursting with happiness. So began a taper of all the unnecessary medication. One by one they were stripped away, with the withdrawals tempered by Lorazepam. Soon there were just three medications left, including Haloperidol, Nicola's mainstay. Every physical test imaginable was used to check out Nicola's physical health. Then came the talk about managing one's lifestyle on Clozapine, such as the numerous blood tests to check white blood cells. This was very important, as Nicola was already on an immunosuppressant for ulcerative colitis, and she did not want to develop agranulocytosis, a serious adverse reaction. This all took several months, and Nicola made a lot of friends in the ward. She understood that she would be there for some time but was aghast at some of the patients who were being trialled on various medications and were still not making progress. While things felt a little rocky for Nicola withdrawing from multiple drugs, it gave me the time to investigate the idea of 'fast metabolizer'.

I found a company in Copenhagen that could do DNA testing. It would tell which drugs would not be effective at all for Nicola and which would be partially effective. It showed that she was an 'ultra-rapid metabolizer' of several drugs, with a poor response to Lithium. The report detailed the clinical consequences, dosing guidance, and risk management, and also covered drugs for every affliction. It was a little difficult for me to decipher, so I had to use some expert help. I felt reassured when the amount of Clozapine was increased to a level four times higher than most other patients—to 900 mg. This showed that the Clozapine level was now in the normal range and effective.

It appears that 7 per cent of Caucasians are rapid metabolizers and require more than average doses of drugs metabolized by CYP2D6 to reach plasma concentrations. The main one which affected Nicola was the Haloperidol, of which she needed so much more than was recommended, and it caused consternation even years later whenever she met former staff. She suffered through many dressing downs over the years, but she could now turn the tables on them.

CHAPTER 24

Final Thoughts on What We Could Do Better

Stigma. Having a child with a psychiatric disorder puts you on the front lines of the battle against stigma. And the nature of your child's illness is likely to determine how hard and how often you must fight that battle. As a society, we now speak openly about depression, thanks to New Zealand rugby greats, but we still have a long way to go when it comes to talking about many other types of disorders.

More support for parents. The process of having your child diagnosed with a mental illness is stressful. Not only do you have to take time off work to take your child to a series of appointments with mental health professionals, but you must be prepared to speak openly about all aspects of your family's life. This is cringe world magnified. It is not uncommon for parents to emerge feeling blamed for their children's difficulties rather than supported in their effort to obtain help for their child. Caregiving is not a nine-to-five job with an hour off for lunch. It is a cruel situation which unravels your existing relationships and makes new ones all but impossible. Things seem to be going well, and you start to entertain high hopes that perhaps she will after all make a steady recovery and be able to lead a more normal life. Suddenly it all goes wrong again.

More resources. To receive the first diagnosis and treatment of bipolar mixed state, I realized that you need to have a lot of time and persistence. However, this proved to be not enough to sustain a mentally ill person. So many other factors play a part. The revolving door of psychiatrists gives the chance that your diagnosis will be once again dispelled and another substituted. Sometimes, your current psychiatrist disappears for months at a time, and you end up at a GP who mostly doesn't have a clue. Or if you can afford it, you go to a private psychiatrist to get continuation of treatment. It is simply that there are not enough public resources. The waiting lists can be horrendous. It is often suggested that therapy is required. Nicola was never offered any kind of therapy. To access this privately, in the form of a clinical psychologist or psychotherapist, up to $300 an hour can be required. Add to this a private psychiatrist for over $500 an hour, and there is someone's weekly salary gone. A counsellor (about $120 an hour) is more affordable, but they will have no clue as to what you are talking about, and you end up educating them for the whole session.

Precision medicine. Mental illness is a complex condition that weaves genetics with environment in ways we do not understand. Our approach to treatment in New Zealand can be hit-and-miss. Years may pass by with many trials of medication and inpatient treatment for the patient, costing the country's health budget a nightmare sum. To hasten the diagnosis and treatment and to rule out other causes, it would be of great benefit to get various tests done which are routinely done overseas.

These tests could be an Obstructive Sleep Apnoea Test which might show the reason for general low functioning or a brain scan (which did show atrophy like a sixty-five-year-old's in Nicola's frontal lobe). Fortunately, there was no dementia, as the scarring was from repeated periods of attacks of bipolar. A DNA report could show response or nonresponse to medications or rate of metabolism of various medications. It is also important to screen for trauma and to have a programme incorporated into treatment planning. Lastly, a dedicated assessment for a personality disorder could be enlightening. All the tests could be carried out in three weeks, and years of fruitless appointments and medications could have been saved, along with thousands of dollars knocked from the health budget. It has always been a puzzle to me as to why in New Zealand, patients can languish in hospital wards month after month, fiddling around with various concoctions of medication, when an obvious answer might be so easily obtained for as little as $600 for a DNA test or $500 for a sleep test. And how much does a night cost in a psychiatric ward? $800? Multiply that by months and add to that the continuing trauma to the patient as they encounter abuse from other unwell patients and burnt-out staff, not to mention their own despair at unending episodes.

Precision medicine is a young and growing field, and if this approach is to become part of routine healthcare, doctors and other healthcare providers will need to know more about molecular genetics and biochemistry. They will increasingly find themselves needing to interpret the results of genetic tests, understand how that information is relevant to treatment, and convey this knowledge to patients. It contrasts with a one-size-fits-all approach.

Clozapine. A final point is to make Clozapine more available for bipolar patients. It may be that some patients are not suitable, but overall in New Zealand, it is discouraged unless you are lucky enough to find a psychiatrist willing to put in the work to obtain it for you. Too much time and effort were wasted by me over the years trying to convince clinicians to trial it for Nicola. I had to pull together statements from at least four psychiatrists and a clinical psychologist who advocated for Clozapine for Nicola and launch a campaign. Although I was very grateful for their input, it still meant that she had needlessly suffered for the past decade.

Today in 2020, I am still aghast that patients are being prescribed the antipsychotics Haloperidol and Clopixol, when it is very well known that these can produce tardive dyskinesia, a permanent disfiguring disorder. Clozapine was a miracle drug for Nicola, and it worked better the longer she took it. After six months, it was decided to further increase the bioavailability of Clozapine by adding in 3,000 mg Epilim.

Today Nicola leads a productive and satisfying life and I continue to advocate for Clozapine for bipolar mixed mood, and broadcast the risk of taking dangerous old style antipsychotics.

APPENDIX

Before Drugs Were Rationalized to Clozapine 2018

Morning

Epilim .... 34 mls (liquid)

Tegretol .... 24 mls

Microlut 2

Pentasa .... 8 Tabs

Haloperidol .... 6 mg

Diazepam .... 2.5 mg

Prazosin 2

Lamotrigine .... 50 mg

Noon

Epilim .... 34 mls

Tegretol .... 24 mls

Haloperidol .... 6 mg

Evening

Epilim .... 34 mls

Tegretol .... 24 mls

Prazosin 2

Olanzapine .... 55 mg

Haloperidol .... 8.5 mg

Diazepam .... 5 mg

Solian .... 300 mg

Lamotrigine .... 50 mg

Kemadrin .... prn

REFERENCES

Akiskal, H. S., et al. (2011). *Bipolar Psychopharmacotherapy: Caring for the Patient*. West Sussex, UK: Wiley.

American Psychiatric Association (2013). *Diagnostic and Statistical Manual of Mental Disorders*.

Ford, J., and Wortman, J. (2013). *Hijacked by Your Brain*. Sourcebooks.

Geller, B., and Del Bello, M. P. (2008), *Treatment of Bipolar in Children and Adolescents*. New York: The Guilford Press.

Demyttenaere, K. (2019). *What Is Treatment Resistance in Psychiatry? A 'Difficult to Treat Concept'*. World Psychiatry.

Sanches, G. D., et al. (2007). *Intensive Care of Postoperative Patients in Bariatric Surgery*. Google Scholar.

www.ingramcontent.com/pod-product-compliance
Lightning Source LLC
Chambersburg PA
CBHW021006180526
45163CB00005B/1910